Dr Sebi Alkaline Diet Smoothie Recipes Food Book: Discover Delicious Alkaline & Electric Smoothies to Naturally Cleanse, Revitalize, and Heal Your Body with Dr. Sebi's Approved Diets.

Copyright © 2020 by Stephanie Quiñones
All rights reserved.

No part of this publication may be reproduced, distributed, or transmitted in any form or by any means, including photocopying, recording, or other electronic or mechanical methods, without the prior written permission of the publisher, except in the case of brief quotations embodied in critical reviews and certain other noncommercial uses permitted by copyright law.

This book is not intended as a substitute for the medical advice of physicians. The reader should regularly consult a physician in matters relating to his/her health and particularly with respect to any symptoms that may require diagnosis or medical attention.

Although the author and publisher have made every effort to ensure that the information in this book was correct at press time, the author and publisher do not assume and hereby disclaim any liability to any party for any loss, damage, or disruption caused by errors or omissions, whether such errors or omissions result from negligence, accident, or any other cause.

Ebook ASIN: B08BZPN5GR
ISBN: 9798657536508

Acknowledgement

I want to thank you and congratulate you for downloading the book, "**Dr Sebi Alkaline Diet Smoothie Recipes Food Book**".

If you interested in learning the latest scientific breakthroughs in fat loss? You are not alone! Millions of people all over the world are trying to lose weight and do so in a safe and effective manner.

What I have done is put together 3 totally *FREE e-books* to get you started on the road to success. These reports won't be up forever, so get them before they are taken down.

It's my simple way of saying thank you for downloading this book. CLICK HERE TO GET INSTANCE ACCESS **or** https://stephaniequinones6.wixsite.com/freereports

Download 3 of the BEST E-books ABSOLUTELY FREE that will help you lose weight, melt off fat, and get in great shape!

Report #1: Top Delicious Fruits for Weight Loss

Report #2: 10 Easiest Fat-Trimming Workouts for Weight Loss

Report #3: Top 4 Tips for Getting Rid of Belly Fat

Dedication

I would like to dedicate this book to Dr. Sebi for sharing the knowledge of the power of Alkaline, Electric Food, and the Medicinal Herbs diet that heals the body and cures diseases. You have inspired me to change my nutrition in my life and make life so much satisfying to live. I honored your hardwork and determination in providing us with the knowledge to overcome adversity. I will not take this for granted and will pass along your powerful knowledge about health and nutrition through the Alkaline and Electric Foods diet.

Table Of Content

Acknowledgement

Dedication

Table Of Content

Introduction

CHAPTER 1: UNDERSTANDING THE MEANING OF ALKALINE
- Importance of pH in the Body
- Health Consequences of Acidity in the Body

CHAPTER 2: THE AMAZING HEALTH BENEFITS OF THE ALKALINE SMOOTHIE DIET
- Best Alkaline Food
- Hybrid Foods

CHAPTER 3: DELICIOUS ALKALINE SMOOTHIES
- Green Alkaline smoothie
- Minty Alkaline Smoothie
- Cherry Alkaline Smoothie
- Boosting Alkaline Smoothie
- Banana Alkaline Smoothie
- Ginger Alkaline Smoothie
- Avocado Alkaline Smoothie
- Kale Alkaline Smoothie
- Cucumber Alkaline Smoothie
- Alkaline Pineapple Smoothie
- Mango Alkaline Smoothie
- Vegetable Alkaline Smoothie

CHAPTER 4: ELECTRIC FOODS
- What is the Electric Food Diet?
- Key Rules of Dr. Sebi's Electric Food Diet
- Foods Allowed on the Electric Food Diet
- Foods that are not Permitted on this Diet
- Electric Herbs

CHAPTER 5: HEALTH BENEFITS OF THE ELECTRIC SMOOTHIE DIET
    Restore your alkaline state:
    Detoxify your body:
    Cure anemia:
    Treat leukemia and lupus:
    Revert diabetes:
    Clears Pneumonia:
    Other Health Benefits

CHAPTER 6: DELICIOUS ELECTRIC FOOD SMOOTHIES
    Electric Berry Sea Moss Smoothie
    Electric Raspberry Greens Smoothie
    Electric Mango-Banana Smoothie
    Electric Sea Moss Green Smoothie
    Electric Kale Berry Smoothie
    Electric Apple Juice Smoothie
    Electric Banana Flax Smoothie
    Electric Green Smoothie
    Electric Apple Berries Smoothie
    Electric Banana Berry Kale Smoothie
    Electric Banana Coconut Smoothie
    Electric Banana Berries Smoothie

BONUS CONTENT: Dr. SEBI'S MEDICINAL HERBAL PLANTS
    Dr. Sebi's Herbal Medicinal Plants
    Top 10 Medicinal Herbal Plants and its recommended Uses

CONCLUSION

THANK YOU

ABOUT AUTHOR

Introduction

Alfredo Darrington Bowman, fondly called Dr. Sebi, was a healer and herbalist who practiced in the United States in the 20th century and 21st century. Some of his works and principles remain through even in these modern times. Dr. Sebi was born in 1933 in Honduras and is an African. As he grew older, he became dissatisfied with some of the Western medical practices and began looking for new solutions to some of the serious medical conditions of the 20th century. After visiting a herbalist in Mexico who healed him of his asthma, diabetes, and impotence, he went back to Honduras. He began his healing practice, and after years of research, he developed a treatment called the African Bioelectric Cell Food Therapy, which he claimed could cure a wide range of illnesses, including AIDS, which was one of the major medical conditions of the 20th century. After developing his treatment, Bowman established his center in Honduras and began to sell his products to the United States. He eventually moved to New York, where he met a lot of legal opposition as a result of his claims, and after a while, he moved to California.

Dr. Sebi's diet was based on the use of natural foods and vegetables to revitalize the body's cells and internal cleansing. Dr. Sebi believed that eating certain foods and staying away from some would help the body to detoxify and achieve an alkaline state, thereby reducing the risk of diseases. He also believed that acidity in the body was one of the major causes of disease infection. While a lot of people criticized his beliefs and practices because they did not have any scientific backing and did not follow any of the medical principles of that time, some subscribed to his beliefs, and he soon began to develop a clientele such as Lisa Lopes, Steven Seagal, Eddie Murphy, John Travolta, and Michael Jackson. In August 2016, Alfredo Bowman died on the way to the hospital as a result of some complications. His teachings and treatment methods have spread across the world after his death, with more people making use of it than ever before.

CHAPTER 1

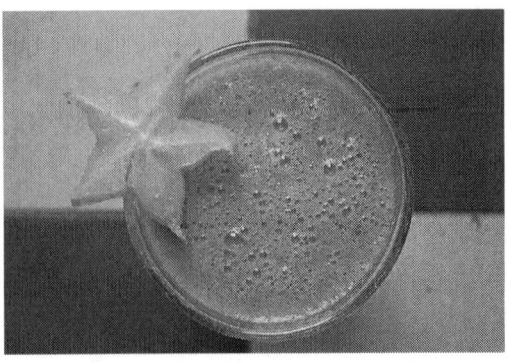

UNDERSTANDING THE MEANING OF ALKALINE

When we hear the word 'Alkaline,' we immediately think about alkaline water that we have heard so much about the litmus paper that we used for experiments in high school. While those do give us an understanding of what alkaline is no matter how little. Alkaline refers to the pH level of a substance, whether it is food, water, the human body. Alkaline also refers to the dissolution of a solution called alkali (derived from the Arabic word 'qali,' which means from the ashes'). An alkali does not have to be a particular substance or material, and it can even be food or water. In fact, the stomach releases an alkaline liquid called bile that AIDS in the digestion of food, and the mixture of the bile with the food and other enzymes in the stomach creates an alkaline solution. Apart from the stomach, the small intestine also has enzymes that work at a pH of 12. Alkaline solutions can be formed through natural processes like erosion and can also be manufactured in a laboratory. Since it is basic, alkaline solutions are used in laboratories to make chemical reactions neutral or basic. It is these alkaline solutions that turn red litmus paper blue as we were shown in high school. Like acid, the level of alkaline in a particular food or substance is measured using pH levels (a pH level helps to determine how acidic or alkaline a substance is). However, determining the strength of an alkaline material requires a little more than pH levels, and this is where a little chemistry comes in. To determine the strength of alkaline, you have to add a universal indicator (a universal indicator is a combination of other indicators e.g., methyl blue) to your substance but when it comes to food or water, all you need to know most times are their pH levels especially if you are on a diet. Before I continue, I must mention that any substance with a pH level greater than 7 is alkaline, while a substance with a pH level of 7 is neutral.

Now that we have gotten that out of the way, how does an alkaline diet work? Am I going to have to work out and give up a lot of the food I love for this diet? An alkaline diet starts with a promise; a promise that by the end of the diet, you would achieve not only your dream body but also rid your body of all the toxins and acids that made your body that way in the first place and by the time you are done, your body will have a fresh start. An alkaline diet is a diet that aims to increase the body's alkalinity and make it less acidic. This diet recommends complete departure from foods such as sugar, processed foods, snacks, dairy products, red meat, and other food items that can increase the body's acidity. This diet majorly focuses on the use of fruits and vegetables to maintain a healthy weight while ridding the body of harmful toxins and acids that had caused unhealthy weight gain. The premise of this diet is that it can alter your body's pH levels in a way that would be beneficial to it by eating certain foods that have high levels of alkaline. Proponents of this diet also claim that following this diet can help to reduce the risk of cancer, kidney stones, diabetes and can also help to improve health and overall wellness. The alkaline diet is about bringing back good old-fashioned healthy eating habits where natural foods were placed above sugars, dairy, and processed food. When it comes to cancer, some studies suggest that cancer thrives in an acidic environment; therefore, when you increase your body's alkalinity, you are reducing your body's risk of having cancer. However, there is still a lot of debate on how an alkaline diet helps to prevent cancer, but one sure thing is that an alkaline diet does aid in losing weight and improving the body's overall function. When starting the alkaline diet, you need to have it at the back of your mind that you would be giving up about 90% of the foods you are used to, and you cannot just order take-outs any time you like during the diet.

You cannot eat any of the dairy products you are used to eating or the chocolates that you adore so much. If you are an early morning coffee type of person, know that you would not be allowed to take coffee or any form of caffeine during the diet, and alcohol is also prohibited during the diet. This diet does a complete reset of the body and restores it to its healthy fat-burning state. Nuts and seeds are also allowed in this diet since they increase alkalinity in the body. Since you are not going to be buying any processed or canned goods during this diet, you would have to cook and prep most of your meals and drinks if you do not want to drink water. Also, there would be little or no need to exercise since your body would be running on a lesser amount of calories than it used to have. This diet is completely vegetarian due to the absence of meat, and it is also gluten-free, so make sure that anything you buy at the grocery store is gluten-free. This diet also reduces the risk of allergies since many of the foods we eat that would result in allergies are cut out as well and, you can do this diet on your own because it is easy to follow, and there are hardly any complications when following this diet.

Importance of pH in the Body

Have you heard of the term 'pH balance' and wondered what it meant? There are acids in our body which are necessary for digestion and other bodily functions and, there is alkaline in the body as well. The body has its way of maintaining pH balance, but sometimes, it might not be able to as a result of the foods and drinks that we take. Most of the foods we eat are acidic, and consuming them in large quantities can cause an imbalance, which would not be good for you and your health. Our cells live and die, and maintaining the body's alkalinity helps the cells to stay alive and function. When our bodies get too acidic, it prevents oxygen from getting to the cells, which can result in the body storing fat in the cells and can lead to the growth of more fat cells, which is the last thing that our bodies need.

If there is no pH balance in the body or if it is too acidic, it could lead to the lungs or kidney malfunctioning, plus, the imbalance could lead to serious medical conditions like acidosis and alkalosis that require medical treatment and not just changes in diet. Maintaining pH balance or a little more alkalinity, allows your body to remain the way it is, and does not put any strain on it whatsoever. Too much acidity or pH imbalance would spell bad news for your immune system as the imbalance would cause your immune system to weaken gradually, thereby making your body more susceptible to diseases. Also, you would begin to feel more fatigued, stressed out, and more prone to mood swings because your body uses essential alkaline nutrients from different parts of the body to make up for what is missing. As a result of the lack of energy you would be experiencing, it would be hard for you to go through the day and carry out all your activities without some form of supplement to keep you going. Like your nervous system, your muscles and joints would also suffer from the pH imbalance. As the acid starts to build up, it would begin to accumulate in your joints and damage your cartilages (the damage done to your cartilages could lead to severe medical conditions such as arthritis). Hyperacidity (the presence of high acid levels in the body) could lead to pimples, blemishes, and other breakouts on the skin because your pH level is imbalanced. Also, the skin could gradually grow weaker and become more susceptible to damage and premature aging.

However, as much as too much acidity is bad, too much alkalinity in the body is dangerous as well, but this rarely happens compared to cases of hyperacidity.

Health Consequences of Acidity in the Body

Acidosis is a health condition that occurs as a result of too much acid on the body fluids, and it occurs when the kidney and the lungs cannot maintain the body's pH balance. When the lungs fail to expel enough CO_2 from the body as a result of conditions like asthma, obesity, chest muscle weakness, chest injuries, alcohol overuse, and the likes, it results in a buildup of CO_2 which increases the body's acidity and the same applies to the kidney. If the kidneys cannot expel enough acid or remove too much alkaline from the body, it would also result in an acid buildup. Apart from the lungs and kidneys, other factors like obesity, dehydration, diabetes, methanol poisoning, aspirin, a high-fat diet, and kidney failure could also cause acidosis. Most symptoms and health consequences of acidosis are popular and can easily be mistaken for something else, but if your body is going through acidosis, you will experience:

- Drowsiness
- Confusion
- Sleepiness
- Headaches that you cannot trace to anything you had done during the day
- Lack of appetite
- Jaundice
- Increase in heart rate since your body is working overtime to make up for the imbalance and;
- A breath that smells a little bit like fruits

These are not all the symptoms, but if you are experiencing any one of the symptoms or most of them at the same time, make sure to go and see a medical professional before things get out of hand. As I mentioned earlier, any food or substance with a pH level that is less than 7 is acidic and for you to maintain your body's pH levels, you can either avoid these foods completely or limit your consumption of them especially when you are not on a diet and just want to maintain a healthy lifestyle. For any food to be considered acidic, it must have a pH level of 4 or lower, and some of these foods that tend to cause more acidity in the body include:

- Sugar
- Grains such as wheat
- Some dairy products such as cheese, full cream milk, ice cream and butter
- Processed foods
- Fish
- Red meat and processed meats like turkey and canned beef
- Soda and sweetened beverages
- Supplements and foods that are high in protein
- Foods that have a high-fat content

Generally, a lot of citrus fruits are acidic in nature and can contribute to the level of acidity in the body. When drinking fruit juice, especially those that are acidic, make sure to keep them away from your teeth as they can cause decay when consumed too much. On a normal day, these fruits, drinks, and foods are okay as long as they are not consumed regularly and do not aggravate any underlying medical condition. A lot of vegetables, especially fresh vegetables, are not acidic, but for your alkaline diet, make sure to avoid sauerkraut as it is acidic in nature. Another thing to note is that most of the fruits mentioned are only acidic in nature, and when metabolized by the body along with other alkaline ingredients, they can serve as blood alkalizing agents.

CHAPTER 2

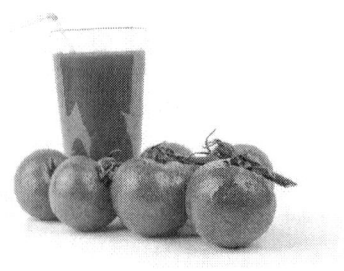

THE AMAZING HEALTH BENEFITS OF THE ALKALINE SMOOTHIE DIET

Since the alkaline diet was introduced, many studies and research have been carried out to validate its benefits. In this chapter, we will be discussing those benefits and some of the scientific research backing them up.

Like most diets, the alkaline smoothie diet also aims to prevent weight gain and promote weight loss. Since most of what you will be consuming are fruits and vegetables, that means that you would be consuming fewer calories than you are used to; also, the diet is low in fat and sugar, which makes it one of the best weight loss solutions. If you want to take the alkaline smoothie without going on a diet, it can also help you lose weight as long as you combine it with exercise and a healthy lifestyle. Another benefit of this diet is that it helps to improve kidney health. According to a study conducted in 2017, most people's typical diet is usually acidic, which can pose a challenge to the health of your kidneys. A lower acid diet can prevent or reduce the risk of kidney disease, and for those who already have the disease, the alkaline diet can help slow it down.

Heart disease is one of the leading causes of death worldwide because a lot of people have poor nutrition, unhealthy lifestyles, and do not do as much exercise or activity as they need to. The alkaline diet can help raise the levels of growth hormone, which helps lower the risk of heart disease also since the diet is low in fat, sugars, and calories help to lower or prevent the risk of heart disease. This diet also eliminates red and processed meat from the causes of heart disease since red meat is not consumed during the diet. Alkaline smoothie diet can also help relieve or lessen back pain (however, it is uncertain whether or not alkaline smoothies help with chronic pain). Osteoporosis is one of the major causes of bone fractures in elderly people and females. The alkaline smoothie diet reduces the amount of calcium that is lost in the urine, which helps to lower the risk of osteoporosis. The smoothie diet is filled with fruits and vegetables, which helps to promote bone health.

As people grow older, they tend to lose muscle mass, which increases the risk of a person falling and having fractures. The alkaline diet helps to promote muscle health by increasing muscle mass, especially among females. Cancer cells thrive in an acidic environment, and since you will be consuming fruits and vegetables that promote pH balance and alkalinity in the body, it can help to reduce the risk of cancer. If you are not on a diet, having a glass of alkaline smoothie a day along with exercise and a healthy lifestyle can also help to reduce the risk of having cancer.

Best Alkaline Food

Alkaline foods are important as they help to bring balance to your body and provide it with a lot of nutrients. Generally, you should be consuming around 60% of alkaline foods and 40% of acidic foods to maintain the body's pH balance. Indulging yourself in excess snacks, sugars, and red meat is not good for your health, and if you are willing to make a change, here are some foods that would be an excellent addition to your diet.

- **Green Leafy Vegetables:** Most of the leafy vegetables around serve as alkaline agents and would be an excellent addition to any diet. Also, they provide essential nutrients that the body needs to carry out its daily functions, and some of the greens you can add to your diet include spinach, lettuce, kale, Swiss chard, celery, parsley, mustard greens, and arugula.

- **Broccoli and cauliflower:** Broccoli and cauliflower not only provide phytochemicals that are needed by the body, but they are also excellent sources of alkaline to your diet or eating plan. Mix the broccoli and cauliflower with other vegetables like beans, green peas, and capsicum, and you would have all the alkaline and nutrients that your body needs in just one bite.

- **Tomatoes:** When uncooked, tomatoes are an excellent alkaline source and still provide a good amount of alkaline to the body even when cooked. They also provide nutrients like Vitamin C, Vitamin B6, and some digestive enzymes to the body. Add some tomatoes to your morning omelets or eat some slices as a snack with a little bit of pink sea salt for some additional flavor.

- **Almonds:** Almonds are great alkaline snacks during a diet and are also an excellent addition to any recipe. The high magnesium content in almonds makes it alkaline-forming, and the healthy fats that are found in almonds make them nutritious and filling. On your alkaline smoothie diet, almonds can be added to the smoothie if you do not mind the texture that it would bring.

- **Garlic:** Garlic is anti-inflammatory and a good source of alkaline, making it one of the best foods you can add to your diet. It has also been proven to help prevent some diseases, improve the immune system, and fight against bacteria in the body.

- **Avocado:** Avocado is one of the superfoods that nature provided as it is packed with nutrients and all sorts of deliciousness. Avocados contain healthy fat, which is good for the body and helps prevent weight gain. Apart from being an alkalizing agent, avocado also helps to improve heart health, and it is anti-inflammatory.

- **Red Onion:** Onions are a good source of Vitamin C and have been proven to have anti-bacterial and anti-inflammatory effects. Cooking it lightly with a bit of healthy fat helps to improve its alkalinity, but it also provides a lot of nutritional benefits when eaten raw.

- **Sea salt and seaweed:** Sea salt and seaweed contain ten times more nutrients than any other vegetable grown on land, which makes it an amazing addition to any diet since they provide a lot of nutrients to any meal. They are also good sources of alkaline and seaweed can be used to make certain dishes while the sea salt can be used to spice up meals such as omelets, salads, soups, and the likes

- **Seasonal fruits:** Any dietitian or nutritionist would tell you that adding seasonal fruits to your diet is extremely beneficial to your health. Seasonal fruits are filled with vitamins, minerals, and antioxidants, which means they provide nutrients that are essential to different parts of the body; also, they are excellent sources of alkaline. Examples of seasonal fruits include kiwi, pineapple, persimmon, watermelon, grapefruit, apricots, apples, and nectarine.

- **Nuts:** Do you like munching on nuts when hunger starts to kick in? Well, it turns out you have been moving in the right direction as nuts are a good source of healthy fat and alkaline. Since they are high in calories, they should not be eaten all the time, and when eaten, it should be in small quantities. Nuts like cashew nuts and chestnuts should be included in your diet plan.

Hybrid Foods

Hybrid foods are the products of the combination of two similar types of fruits. Is it okay to include these hybrid foods in a diet? Do these hybrid fruits and vegetables provide the body with as many nutrients as normal fruits and vegetables? Some people have raised the argument that all fruits and vegetables are hybrid technically due to pollination and other factors; however, that does not mean that hybrid fruits and vegetables are as good as the ones available. Most hybrid fruits are manmade and products of the laboratory. Hybrid foods contain three times the amount of sugar and might not contain as many nutrients as non-hybrid foods so, eating hybrid foods might give your body some problems as it is not used to such high amounts of sugar and mineral imbalance in a fruit or vegetable. Since most of these hybrid foods are grown in the labs and need special conditions to grow, it might contain harmful and toxic chemicals that would not be good for your body. Your overall health and wellbeing depend on your awareness of these hybrid foods and how they can affect your health. When on a diet, it is best to stay away from them and stick to the fruits that you know since the nutrients and health benefits to be gotten from them are guaranteed.

CHAPTER 3

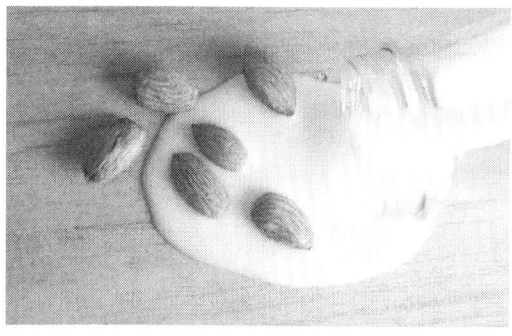

DELICIOUS ALKALINE SMOOTHIES

With all the information you need on the alkaline diet at your fingertips, it is time to go into it properly. In this chapter, we will discuss some smoothies that would be great for your diet and help you start your day feeling refreshed with a good pH. These smoothies are also great for people with acid reflux or indigestion because it contains no acid. Remember that once you start the diet, you could be cutting away up to 90% of what you are used to consuming, but it would be worth it in the end. Also, ensure that you do not have any of the fruits and drinks mentioned in the first chapter because these smoothies are not acidic.

Green Alkaline smoothie

Ingredients:

- ☐ 5 frozen strawberries
- ☐ 1 cup of almond milk
- ☐ 1 large handful of fresh spinach
- ☐ 1 cup of water or ice
- ☐ 1 cup of watermelon
- ☐ 1 small banana
- ☐ 1 teaspoon of chia seeds

Nutritional facts:

Calories: 81kcal
Fat: 2g
Sugar: 8g
Carbohydrates: 14g

When you mix vegetables with berries, your smoothie will become brown, and that is something that nobody wants. So, blend your veggies with the banana, chia seeds, and half a cup of water or ice and then blend the remaining ingredients with the strawberries. Berries are acidic by nature, but we need the antioxidants that the berries supply, and that is why we are using non-dairy milk (almond milk) to neutralize the acidity in the berries so that you can get the nutrients without the acidity.

Minty Alkaline Smoothie

Ingredients:

- ½ kiwi fruit
- ½ a cup of mint
- Cucumber
- 1 banana
- 2-3 tablespoon of honey
- Water or almond milk
- 2 handfuls of Kale
- ½ cup of lemon juice (optional)

Nutritional facts:

Calories: 180kcal
Fat: 4g
Sugar: 15g
Carbohydrates: 10g

Blend the vegetables first before adding the other ingredients. Lemon is acidic; however, the addition of other alkaline ingredients neutralizes the acidity significantly. Also, lemon juice makes the blood alkaline after it has been metabolized.

Cherry Alkaline Smoothie

Ingredients:

- ☐ 1 cup of almond milk
- ☐ 1 cup of ice (if you need it cold)
- ☐ 1 teaspoon of flax seeds
- ☐ 1 cup of seeded fresh cherries
- ☐ 1 tablespoon of raw cashew
- ☐ ½ a cup of chopped beet

Nutritional facts:

Calories: 170kcal
Fat: 3g
Sugar: 10g
Carbohydrates: 17g

Place all your ingredients in a blender and blend until it is smooth with a cream-like consistency. Although cherries are acidic in nature, they are not only neutralized by the almond milk but act as alkalizing agents after the body has metabolized them.

Boosting Alkaline Smoothie

Ingredients:

- ☐ ½ a cup of coconut milk
- ☐ ¼ cup of cucumber chopped or sliced
- ☐ 1 medium banana
- ☐ 1 handful of spinach or Swiss chard
- ☐ ½ a cup of chopped kiwi fruit
- ☐ ½ cup of water or ice cubes

Nutritional facts:

Calories: 130kcal
Fat: 6g
Sugar: 9g
Carbohydrates: 19g

Blend your ingredients until it is smooth. Going on a diet is not easy, especially if you have not done it before as you are cut off from all the foods and snacks that you would normally eat. Keep going, and by the end of it, you would have achieved all the goals that you had set for yourself.

Banana Alkaline Smoothie

Ingredients:

- 1 ½ medium size banana
- ½ cup of blueberries
- 1 large handful of spinach or alkaline greens powder if there is no spinach
- 1 teaspoon of flax seeds
- ½ cup of almond milk
- ½ cup of water or ice

Nutritional facts:

Calories: 155kcal
Fat: 5g
Sugar: 13g
Carbohydrates: 18g

Blend the greens first with the seeds and a little bit of water, and after you are done, blend the banana and other ingredients. Blend for around 1-2 minutes until your smoothie is smooth with a creamy consistency.

Ginger Alkaline Smoothie

Ingredients:

- ☐ 1 cup of water
- ☐ ½ cup of coconut milk
- ☐ 2 cups of spinach
- ☐ 1 ½ teaspoon of fresh ginger
- ☐ 1 medium-sized banana
- ☐ 1 cup of chopped frozen pineapples (or fresh)
- ☐ ½ a cup of freshly squeezed lemon (optional)

Nutritional facts:

Calories: 181kcal
Fat: 2g
Sugar: 7g
Carbohydrates: 11g

If you do not mind the taste of ginger, you can add one tablespoon of it to your smoothie. Blend the vegetables and water until it is smooth, then blend your banana along with the other ingredients. It is best to drink this smoothie immediately after it has been blended.

Avocado Alkaline Smoothie

Ingredients:

- ☐ 1 large handful of Kale
- ☐ 1 cup of avocado
- ☐ ½ a cup of cucumber
- ☐ 1 teaspoon of chia seeds
- ☐ 1 cup of water
- ☐ 1 cup of almond milk
- ☐ ½ a clove of garlic (optional)
- ☐ 1 small handful of spinach (optional)

Nutritional facts:

Calories: 162kcal
Fat: 12g
Sugar: 3g

Carbohydrates: 16g

If you do not like the taste and smell of garlic, leave it out of your smoothie. Blend the vegetables first, then add the fruits along with the milk and garlic afterward, Blend for 1-2 minutes or until it is smooth.

Kale Alkaline Smoothie

Ingredients:

- ☐ 1 large handful of Kale
- ☐ 1 cup of avocado
- ☐ ½-1 cup of chunks of frozen pineapple
- ☐ 1 tablespoon of ginger (optional)
- ☐ 1 teaspoon of chia seeds
- ☐ 1 medium-size banana
- ☐ ½ cup of cashew
- ☐ 1 cup of almond milk or water

Nutritional facts:

Calories: 172kcal
Fat: 9g
Sugar: 8g
Carbohydrates: 24g

Blend the ingredients starting with the vegetables and a little bit of the almond milk or water until it is smooth. Then, add the remaining ingredients and blend for 1-2 minutes until it is smooth with a creamy consistency

Cucumber Alkaline Smoothie

Ingredients:

- ☐ 1 medium banana
- ☐ 1 cup of almond milk
- ☐ ½ cup of cucumber

- ☐ ½ a cup of water
- ☐ 1 handful of parsley or Kale
- ☐ 1 teaspoon of flax seeds
- ☐ ½ a cup of freshly squeezed lemon juice (optional)

Nutritional facts:

Calories: 171kcal
Fat: 6g
Sugar: 3g
Carbohydrates: 17g

Blend your ingredients starting with the vegetables until it has a smooth or cream-like consistency. You can choose not to add the lemon juice if you do not want to.

Alkaline Pineapple Smoothie

Ingredients:

- ☐ 1 teaspoon of turmeric
- ☐ 1 ½ cup of frozen chunks of pineapple
- ☐ 1 cup of cucumbers
- ☐ ½ a cup of freshly squeezed lemon juice
- ☐ I cup of almond or coconut milk
- ☐ 1 teaspoon of chia seeds
- ☐ 1 cup of ice (if you want your smoothie served cold)

Nutritional facts:

Calories: 151kcal
Fat: 11g
Sugar: 10g
Carbohydrates: 14g

Wash all your ingredients and cut them up before throwing it into the blender. Blend for 1-2 minutes until it is smooth and blend with the ice if you want your smoothie cold. It is best to drink it immediately after blending.

Mango Alkaline Smoothie

Ingredients:

- ☐ 1 cup of spinach
- ☐ 1 handful of kale (optional)
- ☐ ½ tablespoon of fresh ginger
- ☐ 1 cup of mango chunks
- ☐ ½ cup of frozen pineapples
- ☐ 1 teaspoon of chia seeds
- ☐ 1 cup of almond milk
- ☐ 1 cup of ice
- ☐ 1 medium carrot

Nutritional facts:

Calories: 232kcal
Fat: 13g
Sugar: 18g
Carbohydrates: 22g

Add water to it, depending on the consistency that you want. Start blending the vegetables with a little bit of the almond milk until it is smooth, add the remaining ingredients to it and blend for 1-2 minutes.

Vegetable Alkaline Smoothie

Ingredients:

- ☐ 2 medium carrots
- ☐ 1 cucumber
- ☐ 2 handfuls of spinach or Kale
- ☐ ½ a cup of apple
- ☐ 1 cup of water
- ☐ 1 cup of coconut milk
- ☐ I teaspoon of flaxseeds
- ☐ 1 cup of ice (optional)

Nutritional facts:

Calories: 90kcal
Fat: 12g
Sugar: 11g
Carbohydrates: 22g

Wash your ingredients and peel your carrots before putting them in your blender. Remove the core from the apples to avoid seeds getting in and blend the vegetables first before putting in the other ingredients. Blend for 1-2 minutes or until it is smooth with a creamy consistency.

This brings us to the end of this chapter, and I am sure that by the end of the diet, your body would have undergone a complete reset. The smoothies mentioned are completely vegan, sugar-free, and do not contain any dairy products whatsoever. During the course of the diet, make sure to stay away from sugar and processed foods so that your progress would not be hindered.

CHAPTER 4

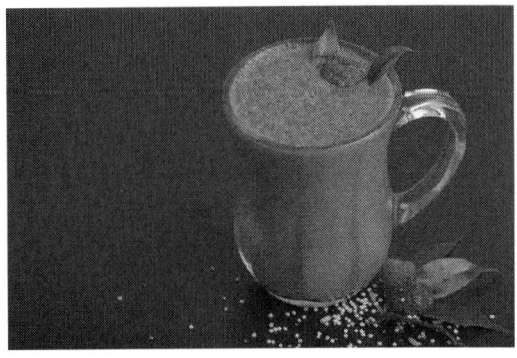

ELECTRIC FOODS

What is the Electric Food Diet?

When we eat, the food that we eat is either healthy or harmful to our body system. Sadly, most of the food we consume do not have nutrients in the proper form for our body to absorb. Generally, most organic foods list nutrients on their nutrients label, but most times, these listed nutrients are not in the proper form for which our body can assimilate. Furthermore, most of our vegetables and fruits are hybrids. These vegetables and fruits simply were made by man. Hybrid foods are high in acidity, which is the opposite of alkalinity. Due to their high level of acidity, hybrid foods cause a disruption in the absorption of nutrients on a cellular level. Therefore, in an attempt to solve this issue of unhealthy and high acidic food consumption by Americans, the idea of electric food was introduced.

Electric foods are foods that are entirely natural, living food indigenous to earth. These foods come from the deep interior of nature, and they remain in their natural state – unchanged by man. The human body is living, and so we need to eat living foods to survive. Electric foods are non-acidic, non-mucus forming, and living foods. Also, electric foods contain alkaline and have an alkaline effect on the body. Unlike other kinds of foods, electric foods can be easily assimilated, broken down, properly digested, utilized, and disposed of by the body. Electric foods are rich in minerals and other rich nutrients that help your body heal from diseases and prevent the outbreak of future diseases. Since the body is created to be naturally electric, it also makes sense to eat electric foods. Now that we understand what electric foods are, the next thing is to explain what an electric food diet is. However, before we proceed, I would like you to take a few minutes to evaluate your health, what you eat, what you drink, and the kind of fruits or vegetables you consume. Having done this evaluation, you may realize that you may have been causing your body more harm than good through what you are eating. The famous Dr. Sebi explained electric food diet had been the root foundation of living a disease-free, non-obese, and addiction-free life. He stressed that the diet was all about minimizing acidity in your food and mucus in your body. Being on an electric food diet means you only eat electric foods that help you develop an alkaline system. This alkaline system built through the electric diet allows your body to fight diseases and prevent the outbreak of future ones. The electric food diet is a culture, a way of life, and a lifestyle. It is not a temporary diet, not something you do only when you are sick or when you want to lose a few pounds. People who are on an electric food diet live a disease-free life. The electric food diet has helped many Americans avoid many of the health hardships prevalent in America today. One importance of the electric food diet is that it helps revitalize your cells by eliminating toxic waste by alkalizing your blood. Electric food entails eating raw foods, sticking to organic and natural foods, and taking a couple of herbal teas and herbal supplements. The electric food diet lacks lactic (diary), uric (meat), or carbonic substances (sugar, salt, and starch).

The human body is naturally made to heal itself, but we can enhance this healing process by feeding it what it needs to operate efficiently and effectively. You don't agree? Or you have doubts. Think about many scratches and scrapes we get that heal on their own without the aid of any medication, orthodox or modern. The electric food diet can be used to restore your body to its natural state and detoxify your body, thereby preventing the outbreak of the disease in your body. The primary bedrock of the electric food diet is education and information. You can start learning about the electric food diet here and then watch out for the change in the trajectory of your health and virtually your life. When you strictly adhere to the electric food diet, you have decided to be healthy and not diseased, be skinny, and not be fat. This one decision is what you need to go from being addicted to being liberated. The electric food diet inculcates in you an alkaline-based lifestyle.

Key Rules of Dr. Sebi's Electric Food Diet

Dr. Sebi's electric food diet has eight main rules that must be adhered to if you want to be healed. These rules practically focus on avoiding animal foods and products, ultra-processed foods, and low protein diet. According to Dr. Sebi's nutritional guide, the following rules are the key rules of the electric food diet:

- ☐ **Rule 1:** You must only eat the food listed in Dr. Sebi's nutritional guide.

- ☐ **Rule 2:** You must drink 1 gallon (3.8 liters) of water every day.

- ☐ **Rule 3:** You must take Dr. Sebi's supplements an hour before medication.

- ☐ **Rule 4:** You are not allowed to take any animal products such as meat or fish.

- ☐ **Rule 5:** You are not allowed to take alcohol.

- ☐ **Rule 6**: The consumption of wheat products is prohibited. You can only consume the natural-growing grains listed in the guide.

- ☐ **Rule 7:** You are not permitted to microwave your food. – Dr. Sebi believes that microwaves kill your food.

- ☐ **Rule 8:** You are not allowed to eat canned or seedless fruits.

Foods Allowed on the Electric Food Diet

Having seen the strict rules of Dr. Sebi's electric food diet, you may be wondering what food you are then allowed to eat. Usually, people think that their food option is limited; well, they are not – Dr. Sebi's electric food diet is basic, simple, and obtainable. Remember that when you feed your body with these foods, you create an internal environment that doesn't harbor disease. Most of the foods, mainly non-hybrid and alkaline-based foods, are highlighted below:

- **Fruits:** Apples, Banana, Orange, Berries (all types, except cranberries), Cantaloupe, Cherries, Figs, Grape (seeded), Limes (key limes, with seed), Mango, Melons (seeded), Papayas, Plums, Peaches, Pears, Prickly pear (cactus fruit), Prunes, Raisins (seeded), Tamarind, Dates, Seville Orange, Soft jelly coconuts, Soursop (Latin or West Indian markets), Tamarind, Elderberries.

- **Vegetables:** Amaranth greens (callaloo, a variety of greens), Avocado, Bell peppers, chayote (Mexican squash), Cucumber, Dandelion greens, Garbanzo beans, Izote (cactus flower/cactus leaf), Kale, Lettuce (all except, iceberg), Mushroom (all except, shitake), Nopales (Mexican cactus), Okra, Olives, Onions, Sea Vegetables (Wakame/dulse/arame/hijiki/nori), Squash, Tomato (cherry and plum only), Tomatillo, Turnip greens, Zucchini, Watercress, Purslane (verdolaga), Wild arugula.

- **Grains:** Amaranth, Fonio, Kamut, Quinoa, Rye, Spelt, Tef, Wild rice.

- **Natural Herbal Teas:** Burdock, Chamomile, Elderberry, Fennel, Ginger, Raspberry, Tila.

- **Oils:** Olive oil (avoid cooking it), Coconut oil (cooking it is prohibited), Grapeseed oil, Sesame oil, Hemp Seed oil, and Avocado oil.

- **Nuts & Seeds (including Nuts & Seed Butters):** Hemp seeds, Raw sesame seeds, Raw sesame "tahini" butter, Brazil nuts.

- **Spices & Seasonings:**

  - ☐ *Mild Flavours:* Basil, Bay leaf, Cloves, Dill, Oregano, Savory, Sweet basil, Tarragon, Thyme.

  - ☐ *Sweet Flavours (Natural Sweeteners):* Pure Agave Syrup (from cactus), Date sugar.

  - ☐ *Pungent & Spicy Flavours:* Achiote, Cayenne/African Bird pepper, Onion Powder, Habanero, and Sage.

  - ☐ Salt Flavours: Pure Sea Salt, Powdered Granulated Seaweed, kelp/dulse/nori – with sea taste.

Note: If a food is not listed above, then it is not recommended. Also, while natural growing grains are alkaline-based; it is highly proffered that you consume only the grains listed above, and not consume wheat. Finally, most of the foods, especially the grains, listed above, are available as pasta, bread, and flour or cereals and can be easily purchased at better health food stores. In any case, foods consisting of yeast or baking powder are prohibited.

Other foods you may be permitted to eat on the electric diet.

Since the electric food diet emphasizes the consumption of nutrient-rich vegetables, fruits, whole grains, and healthy oils, the following are other foods you may be permitted to eat on the electric diet:

- Chia seed
- Quinoa
- Ethiopian teff
- Watermelon (strictly the ones with seeds)

- Sprouts – alfalfa, flax, wheatgrass
- Cabbages
- Coconut

Foods that are not Permitted on this Diet

If any food is not included in Dr. Sebi's Nutritional guide, then such food is not permitted on this diet. Example of such foods are:

- Canned fruits or vegetables
- Hybridized foods
- Eggs
- Dairy (milk)
- Fish
- Red Meat
- Poultry
- Soya Products
- Processed or packaged foods, restaurant take-outs are not excluded.
- Wheat
- Alcohol
- Yeast or foods leavened with yeast
- Baking powder or foods leavened with baking powder.
- Carbonic acids such as salt, sugar (except date sugar and agave syrup), and starch.
- Man-made/hybridized foods
- Seedless fruits
- Carrots
- Broccoli

Finally, many vegetables, fruits, grains, nuts, and seeds are banned on the electric food diet. Therefore, if a vegetable, grain, fruit, nut, or seed isn't listed above, it may not be eaten during the electric food diet.

Electric Herbs

If you have resolutely resolved to embark on this journey to healthier living, then electric herbs and smoothie are for you. Electric herbs serve as both food and nourishment for the human body and play a huge role in detoxing the human system. The lack of proper exercise and proper nutrition in the body results in harm for the body. Therefore, electric herbs serve as a panacea by providing the body with the needed and essential nutrients through vegetables, fruits, and plant minerals. All of them were living products and fed to the human body, which is also a living thing. Some of these electric herbs include:

1. **Red Willow Bark:** Most, if not all, of the commercial aspirins out there today was extracted from this medicinal herb. This electric herb contains iron-phosphate, calcium, magnesium, and potassium. If you have ever heard Dr. Sebi speak of Cancasha, this is the Cancasha he spoke of. This electric herb is used to cure headaches in adults. Note, however – they cannot be used by pregnant women.

2. **Irish moss:** Is an excellent all-rounder rich in minerals and vegetables. It is also referred to as Sea moss by Dr. Sebi. They can be consumed by people of all ages, and also by pregnant women. They are best consumed raw and wild-crafted.

3. **Burdock Root:** This herb, when prepared as tea, provides all 102 minerals the body is made of. Also, this iron-rich tea can be consumed by people of all ages and pregnant women. Additionally, this herb, when prepared as cooled tea, can be used externally to cure all kinds of skin conditions.

4. **Yellow dock Root:** If you are looking for an electric herb for blood cleansing, then Yellow dock root is your best bet. They can be used by people of all ages; however, they are a no-go for pregnant ladies.

5. **Elderberry:** This electric herb is an excellent choice for an anti-inflammatory and antioxidant electric herb. This herb is an excellent source of phosphorus, iron, potassium, and copper. They can be used by people of all ages, and also by pregnant women.

6. **Other electric herbs:** Basil, Moringa, Cayenne Pepper, Sage, Red Clover, Plantain, Dandelion, Oregano, Thyme, and Sarsaparilla.

CHAPTER 5

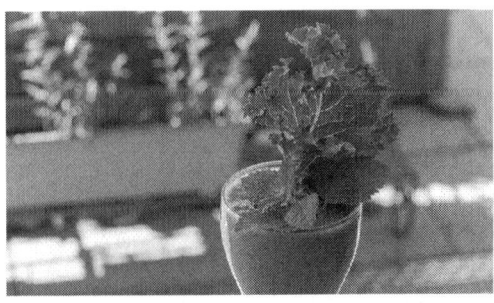

HEALTH BENEFITS OF THE ELECTRIC SMOOTHIE DIET

Like I mentioned in the previous chapter, electric food is natural, indigenous, "live" foods that promote positive changes for a healthy living. Electric foods are leavened with enzymes and beneficial nutrients. The fresher the electric foods you consume are, the more likely it is for you to get these life-transforming and life-giving nutrients. At this juncture, I am assuming that you have commenced your electric food lifestyle, and you are beginning to think, "What exactly are the benefits of the electric smoothie diet?" The answers to the question will be exhaustively provided in this chapter. Keep reading.

One of the benefits of the electric smoothie diet is its immense promotion of plant-based foods. This diet emphasizes the consumption of vegetables and fruits, which have been associated with reduced inflammation and oxidant stress, as well as protection against many diseases. These vegetables and fruits are high in fiber, minerals, plant compounds, and vitamins.

- **Restore your alkaline state:**
  The electric smoothie diet helps improve your body's alkaline state. This diet helps your body maintain its blood pH level. A pH level is how you measure how

acidic or alkaline a thing is. When the pH level of a substance is at 0-6 level, then that thing is acidic. However, when the pH level is 8-14, then that substance is completely alkaline. Note that when the pH level is at 7, the pH level is neutral. Therefore, what an electric smoothie diet does is promote plant-based and alkaline-based foods. This diet emphasizes fruits and vegetables that are rich in alkaline. So when this diet is strictly adhered to by a person, he/she promotes the alkalinity level in their body system and reduces the acidity level. While alkalinity is good for the body, acidity is toxic to the human body system. This diet also helps your body maintain its blood pH level.

- **Detoxify your body:**
  When your body is being detoxified, harmful toxins in your body are extracted. Using the electric smoothie diet to detoxify your body, does a lot of wonder to your body. Since electric foods are high in alkaline and discourage the consumption of hybrid or fortified foods, it is a great choice for the detoxification of the body. When detoxifying the body, you swap caffeinated drinks like tea or coffee for green tea. You, of course, know by now that green tea is an electric food. Fruits and vegetables that are used for the electric smoothie diet are loaded with essential fibers that aid digestion. Cinnamon and fenugreek tea that boost body metabolism are used to detoxify the human body.

- **Cure anemia:**
  Sickle cell anemia is caused by the lack of iron fluorine. You can get sufficient iron phosphate from the electric smoothie diet. The highest concentration of iron fluorine is found in the sarsaparilla root. Other electric herbs with high iron fluorine concentration include: burdock root, cocolmeca, elderberry, nettle, and yellow dock root.

- **Treat leukemia and lupus:**
  By choosing to eat healthier food, eating more fresh fruits and vegetables, eating "live and unprocessed foods, exercising and meditating, these diseases can be healed and reverted.

- **Revert diabetes:**
  Electric smoothie diets discourage the consumption of sugar and starch; hence it can be used to revert diabetes, which is caused by sugar. Consumption of sugar promotes acidity in the body. This acidity, in turn, fosters toxicity and the prevalence of diabetes and other diseases in the body.

- **Clears Pneumonia:**
  Is a respiratory infection that affects your lungs, thereby preventing sufficient oxygen from getting to your bloodstream. The electric smoothie diet discourages the use of dairy products that cause mucus.

Other Health Benefits

Asides the health benefits of the electric smoothie diet highlighted earlier, some other health benefits of the electric smoothie diet are:

- Reduced inflammation stress
- Reduced oxidant stress
- Lowers the incidence of heart disease
- Reduces the rate of cancer diet
- Reduces the risk of heart disease
- Improved diet quality
- Healthy weight loss
- Prevents kidney stones
- Keep bones and muscles fit and strong
- Improved brain function

In conclusion, the electric smoothie diet increases the alkaline in the body and reduces the body's acidity. When the smoothie diet is taken early in the morning, it goes directly into the bloodstream, and the nutrients in the smoothie diet naturally cleanse the liver, kidneys, blood, lungs, and digestive tract.

CHAPTER 6

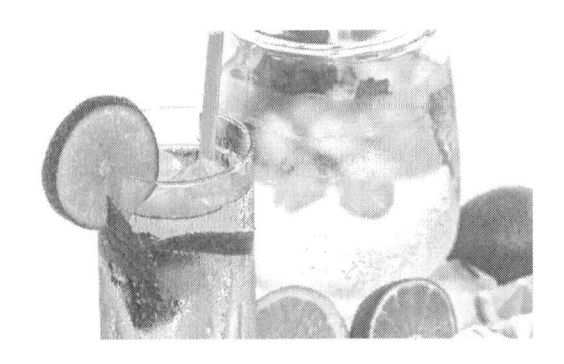

DELICIOUS ELECTRIC FOOD SMOOTHIES

At this juncture, you must have gathered sufficient information on the health benefits of electric food smoothies; it is time to learn how to make those delicious electric food smoothie recipes. This chapter will discuss some smoothies that are ideal for your electric food diet. These smoothies contain amazing nutrients that can help cleanse body organs such as the liver, kidneys, and blood. These smoothies are made with natural, non-hybrid fruits and vegetables – and this is the kind of smoothie your body needs.

Electric Berry Sea Moss Smoothie

Ingredients:

- ½ cup of greens
- One lime (freshly squeezed)
- 1 cup of ice (if you want it cold/chilled)
- ½ cup mixed berries
- ½ banana (frozen)
- Coconut water, 1 cup
- 1 tablespoon of sea moss

Directions/Instruction: starting with the green, blend for one to two minutes. It is better to blend the greens alone first to avoid a brown smoothie. Afterward, add all other ingredients and blend all together until smooth.

Nutritional facts:

Calories: 80kcal
Carbs: 4g
Fat:2g
Carbohydrates: 12g

Electric Raspberry Greens Smoothie

Ingredients:

- ☐ 1 cup of frozen raspberry
- ☐ 2 teaspoons of lime juice
- ☐ 1 cup of coconut milk
- ☐ 1 handful leafy greens
- ☐ 1 cup of ice (if you want it cold)
- ☐ 1 teaspoon of sea moss

Directions/Instructions: make sure you blend the vegetables first before you add other ingredients. Lime is the chief alkaline ingredient in this smoothie. Hence it must be included in the smoothie. Keep blending until all the ingredients have blended smoothly.

Nutritional facts:

Calories: 150kcal
Carbs: 10g
Fat:4g
Carbohydrates: 17g

Electric Mango-Banana Smoothie

Ingredients:

- ☐ ½ banana
- ☐ 1 cup of water
- ☐ 2 cups of greens
- ☐ 1 mango
- ☐ 1 cup of ice (if you want it cold)

Directions/Instructions: blend your smoothie ingredients. Even though the electric food smoothie diet voyage might not be all rosy – you can't eat any of your favorite foods and snacks anymore. However, do not back down, keep your heads up and keep going until you have smashed the goals you set for yourself.

Nutritional facts:

Calories: 155kcal
Carbs: 13g
Fat: 5g
Carbohydrates: 20g

Electric Sea Moss Green Smoothie

Ingredients:

- ☐ 2 full teaspoons of sea moss
- ☐ 2 cups mixed greens
- ☐ One banana
- ☐ 1 cup of ice (if you want it cold)

Directions/Instructions: blend all ingredients until smooth. You can decide to add a few cubes or a cup of ice to your smoothie, and you might not add ice cubes at all – it is your choice to make. However, it is essential to state that some smoothies are better served chilled.

Nutritional facts:

Calories: 162kcal
Carbs: 12g

Fat: 2g
Carbohydrates: 11g

Electric Kale Berry Smoothie

Ingredients:

- ☐ 1 cup of water or 1 cup of coconut or 1 cup of nut milk
- ☐ One large apple
- ☐ 2 cups of kale
- ☐ 1 cup of mixed berries

Directions/Instructions: make sure to blend all ingredients until they have been smoothly blended. For this smoothie, you can use either a cup of water, a coconut, or a cup of nut milk.

Nutritional facts:

Calories: 172kcal
Carbs:24g
Fat:3g
Carbohydrates: 26g

Electric Apple Juice Smoothie

Ingredients:

- ☐ 1 peeled apple
- ☐ 2 cups of steamed kale
- ☐ ½ avocado
- ☐ 1 ½ cups of apple juice

Directions/Instructions: carefully arrange all your ingredients in your blender and blend until all the ingredients have been smoothly blended.

Nutritional facts:

Calories: 150kcal

Carbs: 10g
Fat:11g
Carbohydrates: 16g

Electric Banana Flax Smoothie

Ingredients:

- ☐ ½ cup of blueberries
- ☐ 1 banana (frozen)
- ☐ 1 cup of water
- ☐ 1 teaspoon of flax seeds
- ☐ 2 cups greens

Direction/Instruction: place your ingredients in a high powered blender and blend until your smoothie has a creamy consistency.

Nutritional facts:

Calories: 230kcal
Carbs: 22g
Fat:15g
Carbohydrates: 24g

Electric Green Smoothie

Ingredients:

- ☐ 1 cup of coconut water or a cup of filtered water
- ☐ ½ lime (peeled)
- ☐ 1-inch fresh ginger
- ☐ 1 date
- ☐ 1 handful of greens
- ☐ ½ cucumber (peeled)
- ☐ 1 cup of water

Directions/Instructions: first, you blend your greens with water or milk before you add other ingredients. This is done to avoid a brown smoothie – no one wants a brown smoothie. Now, meticulously arrange the rest of your ingredients in a high powered blender and blend until your smoothie has smoothly blended.

Nutritional facts:

Calories: 200kcal
Carbs: 23g
Fat: 14g
Carbohydrates: 20g

Electric Apple Berries Smoothie

Ingredients:

- ☐ 1 cup water or 1 cup of hemp milk (a cup of ice can also be added if you want it cold)
- ☐ 1 large apple
- ☐ 2 cups greens
- ☐ 1 cup of mixed berries (this mixture may include: raspberries, strawberries, and blueberries)

Directions/Instructions: you must first blend your greens separately to avoid creating a brown smoothie. Afterward, carefully arrange the rest of the ingredients in your blender (preferably a high powered blender) and blend until all of the ingredients are perfectly blended.

Nutritional facts:

Calories: 90kcal
Carbs: 14g
Fat: 11g
Carbohydrates: 22g

Electric Banana Berry Kale Smoothie

Ingredients:

- [ ] 1 banana
- [ ] 1 cup of strawberries (could be fresh or frozen)
- [ ] 1 cup of ice
- [ ] 1 cup of chopped kale

Directions/Instructions: meticulously place the ingredients in your high powered blender and blend until a desired creamy consistency is achieved.

Nutritional facts:

Calories: 171kcal
Carbs: 12g
Fat: 6g
Carbohydrates: 16g

Electric Banana Coconut Smoothie

Ingredients:

- [ ] 1 pear
- [ ] 1 banana
- [ ] 1 cup of coconut water
- [ ] 2 cups of kale (preferably chopped kale)
- [ ] 1 cup of ice (if you desire to serve smoothie chilled)

Directions/Instructions: to get the best out of this smoothie, make sure to carefully place the ingredients mentioned above in a high-powered blender and blend it to satisfaction. Remember that the kale must be chopped to get the best nutritional effect of this smoothie.

Nutritional facts:

Calories: 200kcal
Carbs: 22g
Fat: 12g
Carbohydrates: 24g

Electric Banana Berries Smoothie

Ingredients:

- ☐ 1 handful of watercress
- ☐ ½ cup of blueberries
- ☐ Three baby bananas
- ☐ 1 thumb ginger
- ☐ 2 cups of springs or coconut water
- ☐ ¼ cup of lime juice
- ☐ 1 tablespoon of burdock root powder
- ☐ 6 dates
- ☐ 1 cup of ice (if you want to serve chilled or cold)

Directions/Instructions: carefully arrange and combine all the ingredients into a blender. Then, proceed to blend for two minutes or more. The most important thing is for all the ingredients to be completely mixed into a thick drink. You can add a cup of ice if you want to serve cold or chilled.

Nutritional facts:

Calories: 172kcal
Carbs: 20g
Fat: 9g
Carbohydrates: 28g

BONUS CONTENT

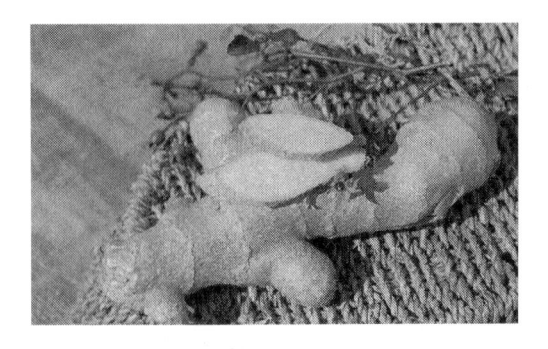

Dr. SEBI'S MEDICINAL HERBAL PLANTS

Dr. Sebi's Medicinal Herbal Plants

- ☐ Basil leaves
- ☐ Turmeric
- ☐ Ginger
- ☐ Mint
- ☐ Cinnamon
- ☐ Chamomile
- ☐ Evening primrose oil
- ☐ Tea tree oil
- ☐ Echinacea
- ☐ Grape seed extract
- ☐ Lavender

Top 10 Medicinal Herbal Plants and its recommended Uses

In this century, we live in a world where manufactured, and processed medicines are prevalent. However, that doesn't mean that herbal medicines cannot be used as an alternative for healing and treatment. After all, herbal medicinal plants are the genesis of how medication started. Also, herbal medicinal plants have the ability to heal, treat, remedy and boost physical and mental fitness or well-being. While it is a known fact that these processed and manufactured medicines have become an integral part of this generation, it can be relieving and soothing to know that we can also approach nature for the power of healing and treatment. These herbal medicinal plants are available as an alternative and complement to our modern health practices and medications. If you would like to add some herbal medicinal plants to your medicinal lifestyle, then I hope this bonus section arms you with sufficient knowledge to start your herbal medicinal plant voyage. Here are ten medicinal herbal plants and its recommended uses:

1. **Turmeric:** Originally from India, turmeric is believed to have anticancer elements and can prevent DNA mutations. This herb can also be used as an anti-inflammatory for older adults who have arthritis. Furthermore, recent studies and research have shown that turmeric is a prospective treatment for various dermatologic diseases and joint diseases such as arthritis. When it comes to culinary functions, turmeric can be used as a cooking ingredient. It is a delicious, antioxidant-rich ingredient to an array of many dishes. This medicinal herbal plant is best consumed when ingested as an herb in cooking or tea. Short-term use is highly recommended – long term use can potentially result in stomach complications. Turmeric has been used as a medicinal herbal plant for over 4, 000 years.

2. **Aloe Vera:** This medicinal herbal plant is popularly known as the 'king of medicinal herbal plant.' Aloe Vera is well-known for its ability to survive in extremely dry conditions as it contains water in its fleshy leaves. Aloe Vera is renowned as a cure to a wide variety of health issues, such as Acne, Constipation, Poor Immune system, Digestive issues.

3. **Flaxseed:** If you are looking for a safe choice for dietary supplements among medicinal herbal plants, then the flaxseed is your go-to. Although subjected to further research and studies, one researcher once asserted that flaxseed could be used to prevent colon

cancer. However, today, flaxseed is recognized as a go-to medicinal herb for its antioxidant effect and anti-inflammatory advantages. Another research claims that flaxseed, when consumed, can aid the reduction of obesity. Flaxseeds are available in oil, flour, and tablets, and can be added to oatmeal and smoothies. For plant-based sources for fatty acids, flax seeds are your best bet. To avoid the toxic effect of the flaxseed, do not consume raw or unripe flaxseed.

4. **Gingko:** Is a key medicinal herbal plant in the Chinese and Asian medical world in general. This herbal plant is the oldest medicinal herbal plant, and the leaves are used by modern medical practitioners to create capsules, tablets, and extracts. While traditionally, ginkgo is consumed as a tea. Studies claim that this herb boost brain health treats patients with moderate dementia, and can influence bone healing. When ingested, ginkgo seeds can be poisonous to the human body.

5. **Tulsi:** In the Hindu religion, this herbal plant has huge religious significance. Besides that, this herbal plant has the ability to keep bacterial growth at bay. Tulsi is known for its strong aroma, and it can be used to: promote longevity, treat cough, treat heart diseases and diabetes, fight stress, and take care of digestion issues.

6. **Mint:** Mint is known for its fragrant, which serves an array of functions. Amongst other things, mint enhances the digestion process and helps lighten your mood. However, for this medicinal plant to thrive, it needs a lot of watering. Another interesting thing about this herb is that, when you plant it in your home garden, its fragrance oozes the ability to chase pets and insects so your home and garden environments will be pest and insect free. Mint is also lauded for its ability to repel cough, boost the immune system, and keep mosquitoes away.

7. **Ginger:** Ginger is widely regarded as a solution to a lot of health problems. In fact, in Indian, ginger, due to its flavor, is an ingredient of Indian foods. Recent research claims that ginger can be used to relieve menstrual pains and cramps. Asides this, ginger can also be used to cure indigestion, cold, flu, asthma, and control blood pressure.

8. **Chamomile:** Chamomile is another great herbal plant that is believed to contain anti-anxiety components. According to a recently published survey, over a million cups of chamomile tea are drunk around the world daily. However, chamomile can also be ingested through capsules, liquids, tablets. If you are looking to treat extreme anxiety disorder cases, then chamomile is a superior solution. Chamomile also has the ability to relieve you from stress and insomnia.

9. **Fennel:** Fennel, also called, saunf, is a medicinal plant with an aromatic flavor. When consumed, fennel is believed to improve eyesight. Fennel seed is a popular herbal plant among Indians – they chew these seeds after eating. Fennel is used to cure cough, control cholesterol, cure, acidity, and improve breast milk supply for women lactating.

10. **Coriander:** Is a medicinal herbal plant that basically can also be used as an ingredient in the kitchen. All its components – seeds, leaves, and powder – have health benefits. These benefits include; improved digestion, treats acne, rich in antioxidants, and cures urine retention.

CONCLUSION

This is the end of the book, and I must commend you, not only for starting this process of learning with me but also for making sure that you see it to the end. However, I must state that it is one thing to learn about a thing; it is an entirely different ballgame to put such knowledge into practice. You must have gained one thing from this book; however, that's not enough – you must also put the knowledge into practice in your day-to-day life. As I have stated earlier in the book, the electric food diet is a lifestyle. It is not a traditional diet that you embark upon only when you want to lose weight. The electric food diet is a diet you have to consistently follow to get your desired results and smash your diet goals. Also, remember to avoid foods with high acidity rates, which can harm the body. Instead, consume alkaline-based foods – they contain nutrients that help cleanse body organs such as kidneys, blood, and the liver. For instance, drink green tea instead of coffee, which is a caffeine product that increases the acidity level in your body. Also, packaged and processed foods are toxic; hence you avoid consuming them. Take-outs from restaurants also fall under this category. Fresh organic foods are the best for your body. They are less toxic and contain nutrients that help maintain the alkalinity level in your body. Finally, remember that we humans, you and I inclusive, are living things, hence the more we consume 'living,' organic or fresh foods, the better our body system. The more we consume 'dead' or inorganic or fortified foods, the more damage we do to our body system. I am sure this book will serve as all the boost you need to start the electric food diet, and I hope you had a great time reading the book as much as I had a great time writing it.

THANK YOU

Thank you for buying my book and I hope you enjoyed it. If you found any value in this book I would really appreciate it if you'd take a minute to post a review on Amazon about this book. I check all my reviews and love to get feedback.

This is the real reward for me knowing that I'm helping others. If you know anyone who may enjoy this book, please share the message and gift it to them.

As you work towards your goals, you may have questions or run into some issues. I'd like to be able to help you, so let's connect.

I don't charge for the assistance, so feel free to connect with me on the internet at:

Join the Smoothie Diet Lifestyle Change Facebook Group

Add Me As A Friend On Facebook

ABOUT AUTHOR

My name is Stephanie Quiñones, an entrepreneur living in the United States who loves sharing knowledge and helping others on the topic of weight-loss, healthy eating, anti-aging, and improving love life.

I'm a very passionate person who will go the extra mile and over-delivers to inspire others to lose weight, be healthy, and to achieve the sexy body they desire.

Stephanie's words of wisdom:

"I believe that knowledge is power. Everyone should improve themselves and/or business, no matter what stage in life they're in. Whether it's to develop a better mindset or to increase profits. Moving forward is key."

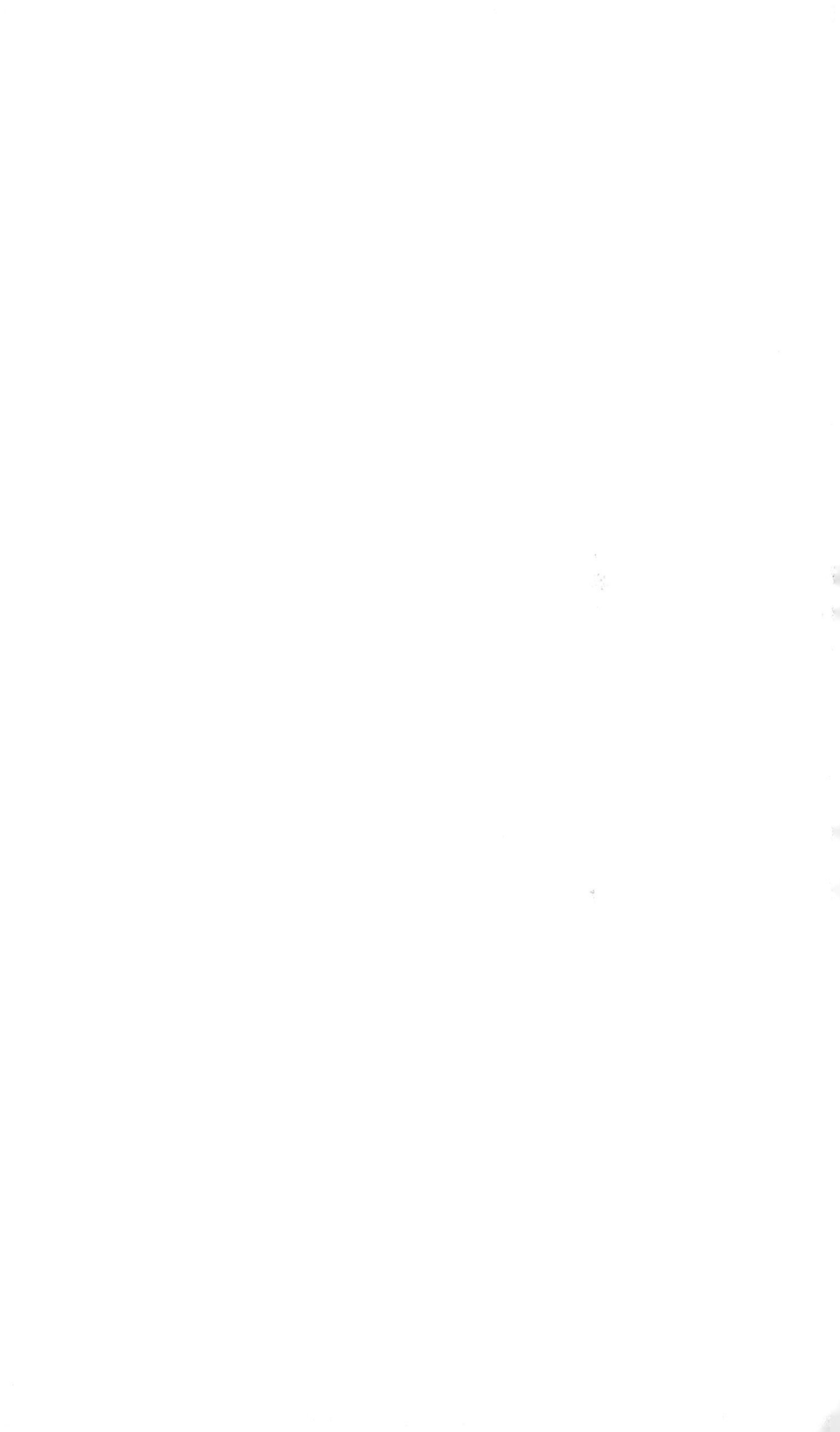

Made in the USA
Columbia, SC
03 June 2021